Sweat, Sleep, Repeat: Harnessing the Sleep Benefits of Exercise

Christopher

Copyright © [2023]

Title: Sweat, Sleep, Repeat: Harnessing the Sleep Benefits of Exercise
Author's: Christopher

All rights reserved. No part of this publication may be reproduced, stored in a retrieval system, or transmitted in any form or by any means, electronic, mechanical, photocopying, recording, or otherwise, without the prior written permission of the publisher or author, except in the case of brief quotations embodied in critical reviews and certain other non-commercial uses permitted by copyright law.

This book was printed and published by [Publisher's: **Christopher**] in [2023]

ISBN:

TABLE OF CONTENT

Chapter 1: The Importance of Sleep and Exercise   06

Understanding the Sleep-Exercise Connection

The Negative Effects of Sleep Deprivation

The Benefits of Regular Exercise

Chapter 2: The Science Behind Sleep and Exercise   12

How Sleep Affects Physical Performance

The Impact of Exercise on Sleep Quality

The Relationship between Sleep and Exercise Recovery

Chapter 3: Improving Sleep Quality through Exercise   18

Exercise Timing: Finding the Optimal Time for Sleep Enhancement

The Role of Aerobic Exercise in Sleep Improvement

Resistance Training and Its Effects on Sleep Quality

Yoga and Meditation for Better Sleep

Chapter 4: Maximizing Sleep Benefits with Proper Sleep Hygiene   26

Creating a Sleep-Friendly Environment

The Importance of a Consistent Sleep Schedule

Managing Stress and Anxiety for Better Sleep

The Impact of Nutrition on Sleep Quality

Chapter 5: Overcoming Sleep Challenges for Better Exercise Performance   34

Addressing Insomnia and Sleep Disorders

Coping with Shift Work and Irregular Sleep Patterns

Balancing Exercise Intensity and Sleep Quality

Chapter 6: Optimizing Your Exercise Routine for Better Sleep   40

Designing an Exercise Program for Sleep Enhancement

Incorporating Cross-Training and Variety into Your Workout

The Role of Rest and Recovery in Sleep Improvement

Chapter 7: Tracking and Monitoring Sleep and Exercise Progress 46

Utilizing Technology for Sleep and Exercise Tracking

The Benefits of Sleep and Exercise Journals

Consulting Professionals for Sleep and Exercise Assessments

Chapter 8: Additional Tips and Strategies for Better Sleep and Exercise 52

The Impact of Caffeine and Alcohol on Sleep and Exercise

Creating a Bedtime Routine for Improved Sleep

The Power of Napping and Power Naps

Chapter 9: Conclusion 58

Recap of the Sleep-Exercise Relationship

Encouragement for Prioritizing Sleep and Exercise

Final Thoughts and Next Steps

Chapter 1: The Importance of Sleep and Exercise

Understanding the Sleep-Exercise Connection

Regular exercise has long been celebrated for its numerous health benefits, from maintaining a healthy weight and reducing the risk of chronic diseases to improving mood and boosting overall well-being. But did you know that exercise also plays a crucial role in enhancing the quality and duration of your sleep? In this subchapter, we will delve into the fascinating connection between sleep and exercise, shedding light on how physical activity can positively impact your sleep patterns and ultimately lead to a more rejuvenating rest.

Sleep and exercise share a bidirectional relationship, meaning that each can influence the other. Engaging in regular physical activity can help regulate your sleep-wake cycle, also known as your circadian rhythm. When you exercise, your body temperature rises, and afterward, it gradually cools down, signaling to your brain that it's time to wind down and prepare for sleep. Moreover, exercise promotes the production of endorphins and serotonin, which are neurotransmitters associated with relaxation and improved mood, further priming your body for a restful night's sleep.

On the other hand, a good night's sleep can significantly enhance your exercise performance and recovery. During sleep, your body repairs and rebuilds tissues, strengthens the immune system, and consolidates memories. Adequate rest also helps regulate hormone levels, including those related to appetite and metabolism, which can impact weight management goals. Furthermore, sleep deprivation has been linked to decreased motivation and increased risk of injuries during physical activity.

To maximize the sleep benefits of exercise, it is important to establish a consistent routine. Aim for at least 150 minutes of moderate-intensity aerobic activity or 75 minutes of vigorous activity per week, spread across several days. However, be mindful of timing your workouts appropriately. Exercising too close to bedtime can leave you feeling energized and make it harder to fall asleep. Instead, try to finish your workout at least a few hours before your desired bedtime to allow your body to cool down and transition into a more relaxed state.

In conclusion, the connection between sleep and exercise is a crucial aspect of overall health and well-being. By incorporating regular physical activity into your routine and prioritizing quality sleep, you can enjoy the numerous benefits that come with a more active and well-rested lifestyle. So, lace up your sneakers, sweat it out, and repeat, knowing that each workout is leading you closer to a better night's sleep.

The Negative Effects of Sleep Deprivation

Sleep is an essential part of our daily routine, just like exercise. However, in our fast-paced society, sleep often takes a back seat to other priorities. The negative effects of sleep deprivation cannot be underestimated, and it is crucial to understand how lack of sleep can impact our overall health and well-being.

One of the primary consequences of sleep deprivation is impaired cognitive function. When we don't get enough sleep, our ability to concentrate, think clearly, and make decisions is significantly compromised. This can affect our performance at work or school, leading to decreased productivity and increased errors. Additionally, sleep deprivation has been linked to memory problems, making it harder for us to retain information and learn new things.

Furthermore, sleep deprivation can have a detrimental impact on our physical health. It weakens our immune system, making us more susceptible to illnesses like the common cold and flu. Lack of sleep has also been associated with an increased risk of developing chronic conditions such as obesity, diabetes, and cardiovascular disease. Studies have shown that individuals who consistently sleep less than the recommended seven to eight hours per night have a higher likelihood of gaining weight and experiencing metabolic disturbances.

Sleep deprivation can also take a toll on our mental health. It has been linked to an increased risk of developing conditions like depression, anxiety, and mood disorders. When we don't get enough sleep, our emotional regulation is compromised, leading to heightened irritability, mood swings, and decreased tolerance for stress.

Additionally, sleep deprivation can have a significant impact on our exercise performance and recovery. When we lack sleep, our bodies have a harder time repairing and rebuilding muscles after exercise. This can lead to increased muscle soreness, slower recovery times, and decreased athletic performance. Moreover, sleep deprivation can negatively affect our motivation to exercise, making it more challenging to maintain a regular fitness routine.

In conclusion, sleep deprivation is not to be taken lightly. It has numerous negative effects on our cognitive function, physical health, mental well-being, and exercise performance. To harness the full benefits of exercise and maintain overall health, it is crucial to prioritize and ensure an adequate amount of quality sleep each night.

The Benefits of Regular Exercise

Regular exercise is essential for maintaining good health and overall well-being. Regardless of age, gender, or fitness level, incorporating exercise into your daily routine can bring about numerous benefits. In this subchapter, we will explore the various advantages of regular exercise and how it can positively impact your life.

1. Improved Physical Health: Engaging in regular exercise helps to strengthen your muscles and bones, improve cardiovascular health, and enhance lung function. It can also aid in weight management, reducing the risk of obesity and associated health conditions such as diabetes and heart disease.

2. Mental Well-being: Exercise is not only beneficial for physical health but also for mental well-being. It has been proven to reduce symptoms of anxiety and depression, boost mood, and enhance overall mental resilience. Regular exercise stimulates the release of endorphins, often referred to as "feel-good" hormones, providing a natural way to combat stress and promote relaxation.

3. Increased Energy Levels: Contrary to popular belief, regular exercise actually increases energy levels instead of depleting them. Engaging in physical activity boosts circulation and improves oxygen flow throughout the body, resulting in increased energy and vitality.

4. Enhanced Cognitive Function: Exercise has a positive impact on cognitive function, improving memory, concentration, and overall brain health. It promotes the growth of new brain cells and strengthens connections between them, leading to better cognitive performance and a reduced risk of age-related cognitive decline.

5. Better Sleep: Regular exercise can significantly improve sleep quality and duration. Physical activity helps to regulate the sleep-wake cycle, promoting a more restful and rejuvenating sleep. It can also alleviate symptoms of insomnia and other sleep disorders, leading to better overall sleep hygiene.

6. Increased Longevity: Engaging in regular exercise has been linked to increased longevity and a reduced risk of chronic diseases. Studies have shown that individuals who exercise regularly have a lower risk of premature death compared to those who lead sedentary lifestyles.

In conclusion, regular exercise offers a multitude of benefits for everyone, regardless of age or fitness level. From improved physical health to enhanced mental well-being and better sleep, incorporating exercise into your daily routine can have a profound positive impact on your overall quality of life. By harnessing the power of regular exercise, you can unlock a healthier, happier, and more fulfilling life.

Chapter 2: The Science Behind Sleep and Exercise

How Sleep Affects Physical Performance

Sleep is a crucial factor that significantly impacts our physical performance. In the pursuit of maintaining a healthy and active lifestyle, it is essential to understand the relationship between sleep and physical performance. In this subchapter, we delve into how sleep affects our overall physical abilities and explore the benefits of a well-rested body.

When it comes to physical performance, sleep acts as a catalyst for optimal functioning. During sleep, our bodies undergo various restorative processes that are vital for repairing and rebuilding muscles, tissues, and cells. Adequate sleep duration allows our bodies to recover from the stresses accumulated during exercise, leading to enhanced performance and reduced risk of injuries.

Furthermore, sleep plays a crucial role in regulating our metabolism and hormone levels. Lack of sleep disrupts the balance of hormones responsible for appetite regulation, leading to increased hunger and a higher likelihood of weight gain. This can have a detrimental effect on physical performance, as carrying excess weight puts strain on our joints and muscles, making it harder to engage in physical activities.

Moreover, sleep deprivation negatively affects our cognitive abilities, such as attention, decision-making, and reaction time. These cognitive functions are essential for athletic performance, as they contribute to focus, coordination, and overall efficiency during physical activities. Lack of sleep can impair these cognitive functions, leading to decreased physical performance and increased risk of accidents or injuries.

On the other hand, getting enough high-quality sleep can have numerous benefits for physical performance. Sufficient sleep improves alertness, reaction time, and concentration, allowing individuals to perform at their best during workouts or sports activities. Additionally, sleep is closely linked to our immune system, and a well-rested body is more resistant to infections and illnesses, enabling consistent participation in physical exercises.

To optimize physical performance, it is recommended to prioritize sleep hygiene practices. Create a sleep routine by going to bed and waking up at consistent times, ensuring you get the recommended 7-9 hours of sleep every night. Create a sleep-friendly environment that is cool, dark, and quiet, promoting deep and uninterrupted sleep. Avoid stimulating activities and electronic devices close to bedtime, as they can interfere with sleep quality.

In conclusion, sleep plays a vital role in physical performance. By understanding the impact of sleep on our bodies, we can harness the sleep benefits of exercise and maximize our overall health and well-being. Prioritizing sleep hygiene practices and ensuring adequate rest will not only enhance physical performance but also contribute to the overall benefits of regular exercise. So, let's sweat, sleep, and repeat for a healthier and more active lifestyle.

The Impact of Exercise on Sleep Quality

Exercise and sleep are two pillars of a healthy lifestyle, and their connection is undeniable. In this subchapter, we will explore the profound impact that exercise has on sleep quality, highlighting the importance of regular physical activity in promoting restful and rejuvenating sleep.

Exercise has long been celebrated for its numerous health benefits, such as weight management, improved cardiovascular health, and increased muscle strength. However, its impact on sleep quality is often overlooked. Engaging in regular physical activity can significantly enhance the duration and quality of sleep, leading to a more refreshed and energized state during the day.

One of the primary ways exercise improves sleep quality is by reducing the time it takes to fall asleep, also known as sleep latency. Physical activity stimulates the production of endorphins, which act as natural sedatives, promoting a state of relaxation and calmness. This not only helps individuals fall asleep faster but also improves the overall sleep efficiency.

Moreover, exercise is a powerful stress reliever. It reduces the levels of stress hormones, such as cortisol, in the body, helping individuals unwind and relax before bedtime. By reducing stress and anxiety, exercise can alleviate common sleep disorders like insomnia, allowing for a more peaceful and uninterrupted night's sleep.

Regular physical activity also plays a significant role in regulating the body's internal clock, known as the circadian rhythm. By maintaining a consistent exercise routine, individuals can sync their body's natural sleep-wake cycle, making it easier to fall asleep and wake up at the desired times. This synchronization enhances the overall sleep quality and promotes a more structured sleep pattern.

Furthermore, exercise can mitigate the symptoms of sleep disorders such as sleep apnea. By strengthening the muscles involved in respiration, physical activity helps maintain open airways and reduces the frequency and intensity of sleep disruptions caused by breathing difficulties.

In conclusion, exercise has a profound impact on sleep quality, making it an essential component of a healthy lifestyle. By reducing sleep latency, relieving stress, regulating the circadian rhythm, and mitigating sleep disorder symptoms, regular physical activity promotes restful and rejuvenating sleep. So, let's embrace the power of exercise and experience the transformative benefits it brings to both our waking and sleeping lives. Remember, sweat, sleep, repeat!

The Relationship between Sleep and Exercise Recovery

In the pursuit of a healthy lifestyle, it is essential to understand the intricate relationship between sleep and exercise recovery. Many individuals focus solely on the physical aspects of exercise, forgetting the crucial role that restful sleep plays in optimizing the benefits of their workouts. In this subchapter, we will delve into the fascinating connections between sleep and exercise recovery, shedding light on the importance of a good night's rest for overall well-being.

Regular exercise has long been recognized for its numerous health benefits. From weight management and improved cardiovascular health to enhanced mood and mental clarity, the advantages of physical activity are vast. However, it is during sleep that the magic truly happens. When we engage in regular exercise, our bodies experience various physiological changes. Our muscles break down, and small tears occur, leading to the need for repair and recovery. This is where sleep becomes crucial.

During sleep, our bodies produce growth hormone, which aids in tissue repair and muscle recovery. Additionally, the restorative processes that occur during sleep, such as protein synthesis, help rebuild and strengthen the muscles, ensuring optimal recovery from exercise-induced damage. Without sufficient sleep, these processes are hindered, leading to decreased muscle growth, increased inflammation, and a higher risk of injury.

Moreover, sleep plays a vital role in the regulation of our hormones. Lack of sleep disrupts the delicate balance of hormones that control appetite, leading to increased cravings and a greater likelihood of weight gain. Additionally, insufficient sleep can negatively impact insulin sensitivity, increasing the risk of developing conditions such as diabetes.

For athletes and fitness enthusiasts, prioritizing sleep is non-negotiable. Adequate rest allows for better performance, reduced risk of injury, and improved overall physical and mental well-being. It is recommended to aim for seven to nine hours of quality sleep each night to optimize exercise recovery and reap the full benefits of physical activity.

In conclusion, the relationship between sleep and exercise recovery is a symbiotic one. By understanding the critical role that sleep plays in optimizing the benefits of exercise, individuals can make informed choices that prioritize both physical activity and restful sleep. By harnessing the power of this dynamic duo, we can achieve our fitness goals, improve our overall health, and enjoy a vibrant and energized life.

Chapter 3: Improving Sleep Quality through Exercise

Exercise Timing: Finding the Optimal Time for Sleep Enhancement

Regular exercise is known to have numerous health benefits, from weight management and improved cardiovascular health to reducing the risk of chronic diseases. But did you know that exercise can also enhance the quality of your sleep? In this subchapter, we will delve into the topic of exercise timing and how it can optimize your sleep patterns, ensuring you wake up feeling refreshed and rejuvenated.

Finding the right time to exercise can significantly impact your sleep quality. While any physical activity is better than none, there are certain timeframes that can maximize the benefits for your sleep. The optimal time to exercise for sleep enhancement varies from person to person, depending on individual factors such as lifestyle, work schedule, and personal preferences.

For those who prefer morning workouts, research suggests that exercising early in the day can help regulate your body's natural circadian rhythm. Morning exercise can boost your energy levels throughout the day, promoting alertness and productivity. It also increases your body temperature, which then drops and promotes better sleep as the evening approaches.

On the other hand, evening workouts can also be beneficial for sleep enhancement. Engaging in physical activity in the late afternoon or evening can help relieve stress and tension accumulated throughout the day, promoting relaxation and better sleep. However, it is essential to complete your exercise session at least a few hours before bedtime, as exercising too close to bedtime can have the opposite effect and make it harder to fall asleep.

It is worth noting that individual preferences and lifestyle constraints play a crucial role in determining the optimal exercise timing for sleep enhancement. Some people may find that working out during their lunch break or in the early evening suits them best. It's important to listen to your body and find a routine that works for you.

In conclusion, exercise timing can greatly influence the quality of your sleep. Whether you prefer morning or evening workouts, finding the optimal time to exercise can help regulate your circadian rhythm, boost energy levels, relieve stress, and promote relaxation. Remember to allow enough time between your workout and bedtime to ensure a restful night's sleep. By incorporating regular exercise into your routine and finding the right timing, you can harness the sleep benefits of exercise and wake up ready to conquer the day.

The Role of Aerobic Exercise in Sleep Improvement

In today's fast-paced world, sleep has become a luxury that many of us struggle to obtain. Although we are aware of the importance of a good night's rest, our hectic schedules often leave us with little time for sleep. However, there is a solution to this problem that doesn't involve sacrificing other commitments - aerobic exercise.

Aerobic exercise, also known as cardio exercise, is any activity that increases your heart rate and gets your blood pumping. This type of exercise has been proven to have numerous health benefits, including weight loss, improved cardiovascular health, and increased endurance. But did you know that it can also improve your sleep?

Regular aerobic exercise has a direct impact on the quality and duration of your sleep. When you engage in aerobic activities such as running, swimming, or cycling, your body releases endorphins - often referred to as "feel-good" hormones. These endorphins not only uplift your mood but also help reduce stress and anxiety, two common culprits that disrupt sleep.

Additionally, aerobic exercise helps regulate your body's internal clock, known as the circadian rhythm. By engaging in physical activity during the day, you signal to your body that it's time to be awake and active. As a result, your body becomes more synchronized with the natural light-dark cycle, making it easier for you to fall asleep at night and wake up feeling refreshed in the morning.

Moreover, aerobic exercise promotes a deeper and more restorative sleep. During exercise, your body temperature rises, and as it cools down afterward, your sleep onset is facilitated. This cooling effect leads to a more relaxed state, allowing you to fall asleep faster and experience longer periods of deep sleep. This deep sleep is essential for the body to repair and rejuvenate itself, leading to improved cognitive function, immune system function, and overall well-being.

Incorporating aerobic exercise into your daily routine doesn't have to be daunting. Start by setting aside just 30 minutes three to four times a week for activities that get your heart rate up. You can choose activities that you enjoy, such as dancing, hiking, or even brisk walking. Remember, consistency is key, so aim to make aerobic exercise a regular part of your lifestyle.

In conclusion, aerobic exercise offers a multitude of benefits, and improved sleep is undoubtedly one of them. By engaging in regular aerobic activities, you can enhance the quality and duration of your sleep, leading to a healthier, happier, and more productive life. So, lace up those running shoes or grab your swimsuit, and let aerobic exercise be your key to a restful night's sleep.

Resistance Training and Its Effects on Sleep Quality

Exercise is often praised for its numerous health benefits, both physical and mental. Regular physical activity has been proven to improve cardiovascular health, boost mood, and even enhance cognitive function. However, one aspect that is often overlooked is the impact of exercise on sleep quality. In this subchapter, we will explore the specific benefits of resistance training on sleep and why it should be an essential part of your fitness routine.

Resistance training, also known as strength training or weightlifting, involves working your muscles against external resistance, such as dumbbells, barbells, or resistance bands. While many people associate this type of exercise with building muscle and increasing strength, its effects on sleep quality are equally remarkable.

Numerous studies have shown that engaging in regular resistance training can lead to improved sleep patterns and overall sleep quality. Resistance training helps to regulate your body's internal clock, known as the circadian rhythm, which plays a crucial role in determining when you feel alert or tired. By engaging in resistance training, you can align your body's internal clock more effectively, leading to better sleep-wake cycles and improved sleep quality.

Additionally, resistance training has been found to reduce symptoms of insomnia and sleep disorders. It can help individuals fall asleep faster, experience fewer nighttime awakenings, and achieve a deeper and more restful sleep. This is because resistance training stimulates the release of endorphins and other neurotransmitters that promote relaxation and improve mood, ultimately contributing to better sleep.

Moreover, incorporating resistance training into your exercise routine can also increase the amount of time spent in deep sleep, which is the most restorative stage of sleep. Deep sleep is essential for tissue repair, muscle growth, and immune system functioning. By enhancing the quality and duration of deep sleep, resistance training can optimize your body's recovery processes, making you feel more rejuvenated and energized during the day.

In conclusion, resistance training offers numerous benefits beyond muscle building and strength gains. It has a significant positive impact on sleep quality, resulting in improved sleep patterns, reduced insomnia symptoms, and increased time spent in deep sleep. If you want to reap the full range of health benefits that regular exercise offers, don't forget to include resistance training in your fitness routine. By doing so, you can harness the sleep benefits of exercise and enjoy a healthier, more well-rested life.

(Note: This content is written for an audience of "EVERY ONE" interested in the niches of "The health benefits of regular exercise".)

Yoga and Meditation for Better Sleep

In today's fast-paced world, many individuals struggle with getting a good night's sleep. Stress, anxiety, and the constant buzz of technology can make it difficult to unwind and relax before bedtime. However, incorporating yoga and meditation into your routine can greatly improve the quality of your sleep, allowing you to wake up refreshed and rejuvenated.

Yoga, an ancient practice that combines physical postures, breathing exercises, and meditation, has been proven to promote relaxation and reduce stress levels. By practicing yoga regularly, you can calm your mind, release tension, and prepare your body for a restful sleep. Certain yoga poses, such as child's pose, forward bends, and legs-up-the-wall pose, are particularly beneficial for promoting relaxation and relieving insomnia.

Meditation, on the other hand, involves focusing your attention and eliminating the stream of thoughts that often keep us awake at night. By practicing meditation before bed, you can train your mind to become more present and let go of the worries and stresses of the day. This not only improves the quality of your sleep but also enhances your overall well-being.

One of the key benefits of yoga and meditation is their ability to activate the body's relaxation response, which is the opposite of the stress response. When we are stressed, our bodies release cortisol, a hormone that can interfere with sleep. Yoga and meditation help to decrease cortisol levels, allowing us to enter a state of deep relaxation and facilitating a smoother transition into sleep.

Additionally, yoga and meditation increase the production of serotonin, a neurotransmitter that regulates mood and promotes feelings of calmness and happiness. By increasing serotonin levels, these practices can alleviate symptoms of anxiety and depression, which are often associated with sleep disturbances.

Furthermore, incorporating yoga and meditation into your exercise routine can enhance the overall health benefits of physical activity. Regular exercise has been shown to improve sleep quality, reduce the risk of chronic diseases, and boost cognitive function. By combining the benefits of exercise with the relaxation techniques of yoga and meditation, you can optimize your sleep and maximize the positive impacts on your health.

In conclusion, yoga and meditation have numerous benefits for improving sleep quality. By dedicating a few minutes each day to these practices, you can calm your mind, release tension from your body, and promote a restful night's sleep. Whether you are a fitness enthusiast or someone struggling with sleep issues, incorporating yoga and meditation into your routine can help you reap the incredible rewards of a good night's sleep.

Chapter 4: Maximizing Sleep Benefits with Proper Sleep Hygiene

Creating a Sleep-Friendly Environment

Getting enough quality sleep is crucial for our overall health and well-being. While exercise plays a significant role in promoting better sleep, creating a sleep-friendly environment is equally important. In this subchapter, we will explore some effective strategies to optimize your surroundings for a restful night's sleep.

First and foremost, it is essential to establish a consistent sleep schedule. Our bodies thrive on routine, so try to go to bed and wake up at the same time every day, even on weekends. This helps regulate your body's internal clock and improve your sleep quality.

Another crucial aspect of creating a sleep-friendly environment is ensuring your bedroom is quiet, dark, and cool. Use earplugs or a white noise machine to mask any disruptive sounds that might disturb your sleep. Invest in blackout curtains or an eye mask to block out any unwanted light sources. Additionally, maintaining a cool temperature, ideally between 60-67°F (15-19°C), can help promote better sleep.

Your choice of bedding and mattress also greatly impacts your sleep quality. Opt for a comfortable and supportive mattress that suits your preferences. Experiment with different types of pillows to find the one that provides optimal neck and head support. Additionally, choose breathable, natural fibers for your sheets and blankets to regulate body temperature throughout the night.

Minimizing distractions in your bedroom is crucial for creating a sleep-friendly environment. Keep electronic devices, such as smartphones, tablets, and televisions, out of the bedroom. The blue light emitted by these devices can interfere with your sleep-wake cycle. Instead, create a relaxing bedtime routine by reading a book, practicing meditation or deep breathing exercises, or taking a warm bath.

Lastly, ensure your bedroom is a clutter-free zone. A tidy and organized space promotes a sense of calm and relaxation, which is essential for a good night's sleep. Remove any unnecessary items and create a serene atmosphere that encourages restfulness.

By implementing these strategies and creating a sleep-friendly environment, you can enhance the benefits of exercise and enjoy the rejuvenating power of a good night's sleep. Remember, quality sleep is a vital component of your overall health and well-being, and with a little effort, you can create the perfect sleep oasis that promotes rest and rejuvenation.

The Importance of a Consistent Sleep Schedule

In our fast-paced modern lives, it can be challenging to prioritize sleep. With endless to-do lists and commitments, it's easy to sacrifice a few hours of shut-eye in favor of getting more work done or indulging in our favorite TV shows. However, establishing and maintaining a consistent sleep schedule is crucial for our overall health and well-being. In this subchapter, we will delve into the importance of a consistent sleep schedule and how it complements the health benefits of regular exercise.

Sleep is not just a period of rest; it is a vital process that allows our bodies and minds to rejuvenate and repair. When we consistently go to bed and wake up at the same time each day, we enable our internal body clock, also known as the circadian rhythm, to regulate our sleep-wake cycle. This synchronization helps us fall asleep faster, achieve deeper sleep, and wake up feeling refreshed and energized.

A consistent sleep schedule plays a significant role in optimizing the health benefits of regular exercise. Exercise enhances our sleep quality by reducing anxiety, stress, and symptoms of depression. It increases the production of endorphins, the "feel-good" hormones that promote relaxation and improve sleep. By incorporating exercise into our daily routine, we can not only enjoy the physical benefits like increased strength and endurance but also reap the rewards of improved sleep.

Furthermore, a consistent sleep schedule helps regulate our appetite and metabolism. When we consistently go to bed and wake up at the same time, our body can better regulate hunger hormones like ghrelin and leptin. This regulation prevents us from overeating, especially late at night when our body is primed for sleep. By maintaining a consistent sleep schedule, we can support our weight management goals and avoid the pitfalls of irregular sleep patterns, such as weight gain and obesity.

In conclusion, a consistent sleep schedule is paramount for everyone, regardless of age or lifestyle. It complements the health benefits of regular exercise by enhancing sleep quality, regulating appetite, and supporting weight management. So, let's prioritize our sleep and establish a consistent sleep schedule to reap the full rewards of a healthy and active lifestyle.

Managing Stress and Anxiety for Better Sleep

In today's fast-paced and demanding world, stress and anxiety have become an increasingly common part of our lives. The negative impact of stress on our mental and physical health is well-documented, but what many people fail to realize is that it can also severely disrupt our sleep patterns. Fortunately, regular exercise can be a powerful tool in managing stress and anxiety, leading to better sleep and overall well-being.

Exercise has long been recognized for its numerous health benefits, but its positive effects on stress and anxiety are often overlooked. Engaging in physical activity triggers the release of endorphins, commonly known as "feel-good" hormones, which help to combat stress and promote relaxation. Regular exercise also increases the production of serotonin, a neurotransmitter that plays a crucial role in regulating mood and reducing anxiety.

When it comes to managing stress and anxiety for better sleep, finding the right exercise routine is key. Different types of exercise have varying effects on the mind and body, so it's important to choose activities that you enjoy and that suit your individual preferences. Whether it's going for a jog, practicing yoga, or participating in team sports, finding an exercise routine that you genuinely look forward to can make a significant difference in managing stress levels and promoting better sleep.

Aside from the direct physiological effects of exercise, it also provides a much-needed break from the daily grind. Engaging in physical activity allows us to shift our focus away from the stressors of life and into the present moment. This mindfulness aspect of exercise can work wonders in reducing stress and anxiety levels, leading to improved sleep quality.

Incorporating regular exercise into your lifestyle can be a transformative experience for your mental and physical well-being. By managing stress and anxiety through exercise, you can enjoy the added bonus of better sleep. This positive cycle of exercise, stress reduction, and improved sleep will create a ripple effect that extends into every aspect of your life.

So, whether you're struggling with stress and anxiety or simply looking to improve your sleep quality, don't underestimate the power of exercise. It's not just about physical fitness; it's about nurturing your mental health as well. Start small, set realistic goals, and gradually build up your exercise routine. Before you know it, you'll be reaping the rewards of reduced stress, improved sleep, and a healthier, happier you.

The Impact of Nutrition on Sleep Quality

In our quest for a better night's sleep, we often overlook one crucial factor: nutrition. What we consume throughout the day can have a significant impact on the quality of our sleep. In this subchapter, we will delve into the link between nutrition and sleep quality, exploring how certain foods and nutrients can either enhance or hinder our ability to obtain a restful night's sleep.

First and foremost, it is essential to understand that a balanced diet plays a vital role in promoting healthy sleep patterns. Consuming a variety of nutrient-rich foods, such as fruits, vegetables, whole grains, lean proteins, and healthy fats, can provide the necessary building blocks for optimal sleep. These foods are packed with vitamins, minerals, and antioxidants that support the body's natural sleep-wake cycle.

One nutrient that has gained significant attention in recent years is tryptophan, an amino acid found in various foods. Tryptophan is a precursor to serotonin, a neurotransmitter that helps regulate sleep. Foods rich in tryptophan include turkey, chicken, eggs, nuts, seeds, and dairy products. Incorporating these into your diet can potentially improve sleep quality.

On the flip side, certain foods can disrupt sleep and should be consumed in moderation, especially close to bedtime. Stimulants like caffeine and nicotine can interfere with falling asleep and staying asleep, so it's advisable to avoid them for at least a few hours before bedtime. Additionally, spicy and heavy meals can cause digestive discomfort, making it harder to fall asleep peacefully.

Hydration is another essential aspect of nutrition that affects sleep. Dehydration can lead to discomfort, such as dry mouth and nasal passages, which can disrupt sleep. It is recommended to consume adequate fluids throughout the day, but be mindful of reducing your intake closer to bedtime to avoid frequent trips to the bathroom.

In conclusion, the impact of nutrition on sleep quality should not be underestimated. By incorporating a balanced diet, rich in sleep-supporting nutrients like tryptophan, and avoiding sleep-disrupting substances like caffeine, we can optimize our chances of achieving a restful night's sleep. Remember, a healthy sleep routine consists not only of exercise and a conducive sleep environment but also mindful choices when it comes to our daily nutrition.

Chapter 5: Overcoming Sleep Challenges for Better Exercise Performance

Addressing Insomnia and Sleep Disorders

Sleep is an essential part of our daily routine, allowing our bodies and minds to rest and rejuvenate. However, for many individuals, the elusive bliss of a good night's sleep remains out of reach. Insomnia and sleep disorders can wreak havoc on our physical and mental health, leaving us feeling groggy, irritable, and unable to function at our best. In this subchapter, we will explore how regular exercise can be a powerful tool in addressing these sleep-related challenges.

Insomnia, characterized by difficulty falling asleep or staying asleep, affects millions of people worldwide. While there can be various underlying causes, stress, anxiety, and a sedentary lifestyle often play significant roles. Exercise, on the other hand, has been shown to reduce stress, alleviate symptoms of anxiety, and improve overall sleep quality.

Regular physical activity helps regulate our body's internal clock, known as the circadian rhythm, which controls our sleep-wake cycle. By engaging in exercise during the day, we can help synchronize our internal clock, making it easier to fall asleep at night and wake up refreshed in the morning.

Furthermore, exercise has been found to increase the production of endorphins, our brain's feel-good chemicals. These endorphins not only boost our mood but also promote relaxation and reduce feelings of pain or discomfort, making it easier to drift into a peaceful slumber.

In addition to improving sleep quality, exercise has also been shown to alleviate symptoms of sleep disorders such as sleep apnea and restless leg syndrome. By strengthening the muscles and improving overall fitness levels, exercise can help reduce the frequency and intensity of these disruptive sleep interruptions.

While exercise can undoubtedly benefit those struggling with insomnia and sleep disorders, it is essential to find the right balance. Vigorous exercise close to bedtime may stimulate the body and make it harder to fall asleep. Therefore, it is recommended to engage in moderate-intensity exercise earlier in the day, allowing the body ample time to wind down before bedtime.

In conclusion, the relationship between regular exercise and improved sleep quality is a powerful one. By incorporating physical activity into our daily routine, we can address insomnia and sleep disorders, promoting better overall health and well-being. Whether it's a brisk walk, a yoga session, or a fun group class, finding an exercise that suits our preferences and lifestyle can be the key to unlocking the restful sleep we all deserve.

Coping with Shift Work and Irregular Sleep Patterns

Shift work and irregular sleep patterns can significantly disrupt our body's natural sleep-wake cycle, leading to a host of health issues and challenges. Whether you work night shifts, rotating shifts, or irregular hours, it is essential to find strategies to cope with these disruptions and prioritize quality sleep. In this subchapter, we will explore effective ways to manage shift work and irregular sleep patterns, ensuring that your health and well-being remain a priority.

One of the most crucial aspects of coping with shift work is establishing a consistent sleep routine. Try to go to bed and wake up at the same time every day, even on your days off. This consistency helps regulate your body's internal clock and promotes better sleep quality. Additionally, create a sleep-friendly environment by keeping your bedroom cool, dark, and quiet. Invest in blackout curtains, earplugs, or a white noise machine to block out any disturbances that may occur during your designated sleep time.

Another strategy to cope with shift work is to optimize your exposure to natural light. Exposure to bright light during the day can help regulate your body's circadian rhythm, making it easier to fall asleep when needed. If you work nights, try to get outside and soak up some sunlight before starting your shift. On the other hand, when it's time to sleep, use blackout curtains or wear an eye mask to block out sunlight and create a dark environment.

Managing your caffeine intake is also crucial when dealing with shift work and irregular sleep patterns. While caffeine can provide a temporary energy boost, it can also disrupt your sleep. Avoid consuming caffeine within a few hours of your designated sleep time to ensure that it doesn't interfere with your ability to fall asleep and maintain a restful sleep throughout the night.

Lastly, prioritize self-care and stress management techniques to help mitigate the challenges of irregular sleep patterns. Engage in regular exercise, such as jogging, yoga, or swimming, to reduce stress levels and promote better sleep. Incorporate relaxation techniques into your routine, such as meditation or deep breathing exercises, to calm your mind and prepare it for restful sleep.

By implementing these coping strategies, you can minimize the negative impact of shift work and irregular sleep patterns on your overall health. Remember, everyone's sleep needs are unique, so it may take some trial and error to find the strategies that work best for you. Prioritize your sleep, and you'll reap the benefits of improved energy, focus, and overall well-being.

Balancing Exercise Intensity and Sleep Quality

Exercise is a powerful tool that can enhance our physical and mental well-being, providing a wide range of health benefits. From weight management to improved cardiovascular health, the advantages of regular physical activity are well-documented. However, it is essential to strike a balance between exercise intensity and sleep quality in order to fully harness these benefits.

Many individuals, driven by the desire to achieve their fitness goals, push themselves to the limits during their workouts. While high-intensity exercise can be effective in improving fitness levels, it can also have a negative impact on sleep quality. Intense workouts elevate the heart rate, increase adrenaline levels, and stimulate the release of endorphins, making it difficult for the body to relax and unwind in preparation for sleep.

To optimize both exercise benefits and sleep quality, it is crucial to find the right balance. Moderate-intensity workouts, such as brisk walking, cycling, or swimming, can provide an effective workout while minimizing the disruption to sleep patterns. These types of exercises elevate the heart rate without overwhelming the body, allowing for a smoother transition into restful sleep.

Timing also plays a significant role in balancing exercise intensity and sleep quality. Exercising too close to bedtime can interfere with the body's natural wind-down process, making it harder to fall asleep. It is recommended to finish exercising at least two to three hours before bedtime, allowing the body to cool down and return to its normal state before sleep.

Furthermore, incorporating relaxation techniques into your exercise routine can have a positive impact on sleep quality. Practices such as yoga, tai chi, or gentle stretching can help calm the mind and relax the body, promoting a more restful sleep.

Finally, it is important to listen to your body and give it the rest it needs. Overtraining or neglecting rest days can lead to fatigue, muscle soreness, and even sleep disturbances. Rest and recovery days are crucial for the body to repair and rejuvenate, ensuring a healthy balance between exercise and sleep.

In conclusion, regular exercise is undoubtedly beneficial for our overall health and well-being. However, finding the right balance between exercise intensity and sleep quality is essential to fully harness these benefits. By incorporating moderate-intensity workouts, allowing ample time between exercise and bedtime, incorporating relaxation techniques, and prioritizing rest and recovery, we can strike a harmonious balance between exercise and sleep, reaping the rewards of both. So let's remember, sweat it out, get a good night's sleep, and repeat for a healthier and happier life.

Chapter 6: Optimizing Your Exercise Routine for Better Sleep

Designing an Exercise Program for Sleep Enhancement

A good night's sleep is essential for overall health and well-being. It not only rejuvenates the body but also enhances cognitive function, mood, and productivity. While there are numerous factors that contribute to a good night's sleep, regular exercise has been proven to be one of the most effective ways to improve sleep quality. In this subchapter, we will explore how to design an exercise program specifically aimed at enhancing sleep.

When it comes to designing an exercise program for sleep enhancement, it is important to consider the intensity, duration, and timing of your workouts. Aim for moderate to high-intensity exercises such as jogging, cycling, or swimming. These activities increase the production of endorphins, which promote relaxation and reduce stress levels. Engaging in cardiovascular exercises for at least 30 minutes a day, five days a week, can significantly improve sleep quality.

Additionally, incorporating strength training exercises into your routine can have a positive impact on sleep. Strength training not only strengthens muscles but also improves bone density and overall physical health. Aim to include resistance exercises at least two days a week, targeting major muscle groups such as the legs, arms, chest, back, and core.

Timing is crucial when it comes to exercise and sleep. Avoid exercising too close to bedtime, as the increased heart rate and adrenaline levels can make it difficult to fall asleep. Ideally, schedule your workouts in the morning or early afternoon. This will give your body enough time to wind down before bedtime, promoting a more restful night's sleep.

In addition to regular exercise, it is important to establish a bedtime routine that promotes relaxation. This can include activities such as reading a book, taking a warm bath, or practicing mindfulness meditation. By combining exercise with a calming bedtime routine, you can create the optimal conditions for a good night's sleep.

In conclusion, designing an exercise program for sleep enhancement involves incorporating both cardiovascular and strength training exercises into your routine. It is important to strike a balance between intensity, duration, and timing to maximize the benefits on sleep quality. Remember to establish a bedtime routine that promotes relaxation to further optimize your sleep. By making exercise a priority in your daily life, you can harness its sleep benefits and enjoy improved overall health and well-being.

Disclaimer: This content is for informational purposes only. Consult with a healthcare professional before starting any exercise program.

Incorporating Cross-Training and Variety into Your Workout

Exercise is a crucial aspect of maintaining a healthy lifestyle. Regular physical activity offers numerous health benefits, including weight management, improved cardiovascular health, enhanced mood, and increased energy levels. However, many individuals find themselves stuck in monotonous workout routines, which can lead to a lack of motivation and boredom. To combat this, it is essential to incorporate cross-training and variety into your exercise regimen.

Cross-training involves combining different types of exercises to work various muscle groups and improve overall fitness. This approach not only prevents overuse injuries but also helps break through plateaus and keeps your workouts exciting and engaging. By adding variety to your routine, you challenge your body in new ways, leading to better results.

One effective way to incorporate cross-training is to alternate between cardio exercises and strength training. For instance, you could engage in high-intensity interval training (HIIT) one day, focusing on cardiovascular endurance, and then switch to weightlifting to build muscle strength the next day. This combination not only improves your overall fitness but also prevents your body from adapting to a single type of exercise.

In addition to cross-training, introducing variety into your workouts can further enhance the health benefits you gain. Trying new activities or exercises not only keeps your mind engaged but also challenges your body in different ways. You might consider participating in group fitness classes like Zumba, yoga, or kickboxing to add excitement and social interaction to your routine. Alternatively, outdoor activities such as hiking, swimming, or cycling can provide a change of scenery while keeping you active.

Another approach to incorporating variety is to switch up the intensity, duration, or frequency of your workouts. For example, you could increase the resistance or speed during your strength training sessions, or lengthen the duration of your cardio workouts. By constantly challenging yourself, you ensure continuous progress and avoid hitting a plateau.

Remember, the key to reaping the full health benefits of regular exercise lies in keeping your routine fresh and exciting. Incorporating cross-training and variety into your workouts not only prevents boredom but also maximizes your fitness gains. So, lace up your sneakers, try new activities, and keep your body guessing – the possibilities are endless!

The Role of Rest and Recovery in Sleep Improvement

In our fast-paced and demanding world, it is easy to overlook the importance of rest and recovery, especially when it comes to our sleep. However, understanding the role that rest and recovery play in sleep improvement is crucial for maintaining optimal health and reaping the benefits of regular exercise. In this subchapter, we will delve into the significance of rest and recovery in achieving a good night's sleep.

Rest and recovery are essential components of the sleep-wake cycle. When we exercise, our bodies undergo physical stress and strain, which can lead to muscle fatigue and the release of stress hormones. Rest and recovery help our bodies repair and replenish themselves, allowing us to bounce back stronger. This process is particularly important for sleep improvement, as it enables our bodies to relax and rejuvenate during sleep.

One of the key ways rest and recovery contribute to better sleep is through the regulation of our circadian rhythm. Our circadian rhythm is our body's internal clock, which helps regulate our sleep-wake cycle. Regular exercise can help synchronize our circadian rhythm, promoting a more consistent sleep pattern. However, without adequate rest and recovery, our bodies may struggle to maintain this rhythm, leading to disrupted sleep.

Furthermore, rest and recovery are crucial for reducing the risk of sleep disorders. Conditions such as insomnia, sleep apnea, and restless leg syndrome can all be exacerbated by a lack of rest and recovery. By allowing our bodies the time they need to repair and replenish, we can minimize the likelihood of developing these sleep disorders and improve our overall sleep quality.

Rest and recovery also play a significant role in mental health and well-being. When we exercise, our brains release endorphins, which are chemicals that promote feelings of happiness and relaxation. Rest and recovery allow these endorphins to dissipate, helping us achieve a calm and relaxed state conducive to better sleep. Additionally, rest and recovery provide an opportunity for our minds to unwind, reducing stress and anxiety levels, and promoting a more restful sleep.

In conclusion, rest and recovery are integral components of sleep improvement. By prioritizing adequate rest and recovery, we can regulate our circadian rhythm, reduce the risk of sleep disorders, and enhance our mental well-being. Whether you are a fitness enthusiast or someone looking to improve their sleep, understanding and implementing strategies for rest and recovery will undoubtedly contribute to your overall well-being. So, take the time to rest, recover, and reap the benefits of a good night's sleep.

Chapter 7: Tracking and Monitoring Sleep and Exercise Progress

Utilizing Technology for Sleep and Exercise Tracking

In today's fast-paced world, where time is always a constraint, it can be challenging to maintain a healthy lifestyle. However, technology has come to our rescue by offering innovative solutions to track our sleep and exercise routines. These advancements have made it easier than ever to stay on top of our fitness goals and achieve a better balance between our physical well-being and our hectic schedules.

Sleep and exercise are two pillars of a healthy lifestyle, and they go hand in hand. Regular exercise not only helps improve our physical fitness but also promotes better sleep quality. On the other hand, quality sleep allows our bodies to recover and rejuvenate, ensuring we have the energy and motivation to engage in physical activities. Understanding the intricate connection between sleep and exercise is crucial for optimal well-being.

With the advent of wearable technology and smartphone applications, tracking and monitoring our sleep and exercise patterns has become effortless. These devices and apps offer a comprehensive overview of our daily activities, including the duration, intensity, and quality of our workouts, as well as the duration and quality of our sleep. This data can be immensely valuable in fine-tuning our routines, setting realistic goals, and staying motivated.

Sleep trackers, for instance, monitor our sleep cycles, providing insights into the quality of our sleep. They can detect how long it takes us to fall asleep, how often we wake up during the night, and the amount of deep and REM sleep we experience. Armed with this information, we can identify any sleep disturbances or patterns that may hinder our rest and take appropriate measures to improve our sleep hygiene.

Exercise tracking technology, on the other hand, allows us to monitor our workouts, whether it's running, swimming, cycling, or any other form of physical activity. These devices can track our heart rate, distance covered, speed, and even the number of calories burned. By analyzing this data, we can make informed decisions about our exercise routines, ensuring we're challenging ourselves enough while avoiding overexertion.

Moreover, many of these sleep and exercise tracking technologies offer additional features like personalized coaching, goal setting, and social connectivity. They enable us to connect with like-minded individuals, participate in challenges, and share our achievements, fostering a sense of community and motivation.

In conclusion, technology has revolutionized the way we approach sleep and exercise. The ability to track and monitor our sleep and exercise routines has empowered individuals from all walks of life to take charge of their well-being. By utilizing these advancements, we can optimize our sleep and exercise habits, ultimately leading to a healthier and more balanced lifestyle. So, let's embrace the power of technology and unlock the full potential of our sleep and exercise routines for a happier and healthier life.

The Benefits of Sleep and Exercise Journals

Keeping a sleep and exercise journal can be a powerful tool in achieving your health and fitness goals. In the fast-paced world we live in, it is easy to neglect our sleep and exercise routines. However, understanding the benefits of maintaining these habits can motivate us to prioritize them in our lives. By using a sleep and exercise journal, you can track your progress, identify patterns, and make necessary adjustments to optimize your overall well-being.

One of the key benefits of using a sleep journal is the ability to monitor your sleep patterns. By recording the time you go to bed, the duration of your sleep, and any disruptions during the night, you can identify any factors that may be affecting the quality of your sleep. This information is crucial in understanding your individual sleep needs and making adjustments to improve your sleep hygiene. A sleep journal can also help you identify any external factors, such as caffeine intake or screen time before bed, that may be negatively impacting your sleep. With this knowledge, you can make informed decisions to create a more restful sleep environment.

Similarly, an exercise journal can provide valuable insights into your fitness journey. By recording your exercise routine, including the type of activity, duration, and intensity, you can track your progress over time. This allows you to set realistic goals and monitor your improvement. Additionally, an exercise journal can help you identify patterns in your energy levels and performance. For example, you may notice that you feel more energized and perform better after a certain type of exercise or at a specific time of day. Armed with this knowledge, you can structure your exercise routine to optimize your workouts and achieve better results.

Furthermore, a sleep and exercise journal can help you identify the connection between these two fundamental aspects of your health. By tracking your sleep and exercise habits side by side, you may notice a correlation between the quality of your sleep and your exercise performance. For instance, you may find that on days when you have a restful night's sleep, you are more motivated and have more energy to engage in physical activity. Conversely, poor sleep may result in decreased exercise performance. Recognizing this connection can help you prioritize sleep as an essential component of your fitness routine.

In conclusion, keeping a sleep and exercise journal offers numerous benefits to individuals of all ages and fitness levels. By tracking and analyzing your sleep and exercise patterns, you can gain valuable insights into your overall well-being. These journals will help you make informed decisions to optimize your sleep quality, exercise routine, and ultimately, your health. So, grab a journal and start harnessing the sleep benefits of exercise today!

Consulting Professionals for Sleep and Exercise Assessments

In the quest for optimal health and well-being, many individuals are turning to regular exercise as a means to achieve their goals. The health benefits of engaging in physical activity are well-documented, ranging from weight management and cardiovascular health to improved mood and mental clarity. However, it is important to recognize that exercise alone is not the sole factor in achieving overall well-being. Sleep, an often overlooked aspect of health, plays a crucial role in our physical and mental rejuvenation.

For those seeking to maximize the benefits of exercise through adequate sleep, consulting professionals for sleep and exercise assessments can prove incredibly valuable. These experts possess the knowledge and expertise to evaluate various factors that may be affecting an individual's sleep quality and exercise performance. By understanding the unique needs and circumstances of each individual, they can provide tailored recommendations and guidance for optimal results.

Sleep assessments conducted by professionals involve a comprehensive evaluation of an individual's sleep patterns, sleep environment, and overall sleep hygiene. They may utilize tools such as sleep diaries, questionnaires, and even wearable devices to gather data. By analyzing this information, professionals can identify any underlying sleep disorders or disturbances that may be hindering quality sleep. They can then provide targeted interventions or refer individuals to specialized sleep clinics if necessary.

In addition to sleep assessments, consulting professionals can also conduct exercise assessments to evaluate an individual's current fitness level and exercise routine. These assessments may involve measurements of cardiovascular fitness, muscular strength, and flexibility. By understanding an individual's baseline fitness, professionals can design personalized exercise programs that cater to their specific needs and goals. They can also address any potential limitations or concerns, ensuring a safe and effective exercise regimen.

By combining the expertise of sleep and exercise professionals, individuals can optimize their overall well-being. The knowledge gained from these assessments can empower individuals to make informed decisions about their lifestyle choices, leading to improved sleep quality, enhanced exercise performance, and ultimately, a healthier and happier life.

Whether you are a fitness enthusiast, an athlete, or simply someone looking to improve your overall health, consulting professionals for sleep and exercise assessments can be a game-changer. These experts can offer valuable insights, guidance, and support to help you achieve the full potential of your exercise routine and reap the benefits of quality sleep. Don't overlook the importance of these assessments on your journey towards a healthier, more balanced lifestyle.

Chapter 8: Additional Tips and Strategies for Better Sleep and Exercise

The Impact of Caffeine and Alcohol on Sleep and Exercise

In our modern, fast-paced society, many individuals rely on caffeine to jumpstart their mornings and alcohol to wind down after a long day. However, what we consume can have a significant impact on our sleep patterns and ultimately affect our ability to exercise effectively. In this subchapter, we will explore the effects of caffeine and alcohol on sleep and exercise, shedding light on the importance of mindful consumption for maximizing the health benefits of regular exercise.

Caffeine, commonly found in coffee, tea, energy drinks, and even some medications, acts as a stimulant that can enhance alertness and improve athletic performance. However, consuming caffeine too close to bedtime can disrupt sleep patterns, making it difficult to fall asleep and achieve the restorative sleep necessary for optimal exercise recovery. Caffeine can also increase heart rate and blood pressure, potentially affecting cardiovascular health. It is recommended to limit caffeine intake, especially in the evening, to ensure a good night's sleep and maintain a balanced exercise routine.

Similarly, alcohol consumption can have detrimental effects on both sleep and exercise. While alcohol may initially make you feel drowsy and aid in falling asleep faster, it disrupts the sleep cycle, leading to fragmented and poor-quality sleep. This can leave you feeling groggy and fatigued the next day, making it harder to engage in regular exercise. Alcohol also dehydrates the body, impairs muscle recovery, and hinders athletic performance. It is advisable to moderate alcohol consumption and allow ample time for the body to metabolize it before engaging in physical activity or going to bed.

To harness the sleep benefits of exercise fully, it is vital to adopt mindful consumption habits regarding caffeine and alcohol. Limiting caffeine intake to the mornings or early afternoon can help ensure a restful night's sleep and support exercise performance. Likewise, consuming alcohol in moderation and allowing sufficient time for it to leave the system before exercising or going to bed can optimize both sleep and exercise outcomes.

In conclusion, the impact of caffeine and alcohol on sleep and exercise cannot be overlooked. Mindful consumption is crucial for reaping the health benefits of regular exercise. By being aware of the effects of caffeine and alcohol on our sleep patterns and physical performance, we can make informed choices that support our overall well-being. So, let's prioritize sleep, exercise, and responsible consumption to maintain a healthy and balanced lifestyle.

Creating a Bedtime Routine for Improved Sleep

Sleep is an essential component of our overall health and well-being. It plays a crucial role in repairing and rejuvenating our bodies, improving our mood, and enhancing cognitive function. However, in today's fast-paced world, many people struggle with getting quality sleep. This is where creating a bedtime routine can make a significant difference.

Whether you are an athlete, a busy professional, a parent, or someone looking to improve their sleep, establishing a bedtime routine can help you fall asleep faster, stay asleep longer, and wake up feeling refreshed and energized. In this subchapter, we will explore the importance of a bedtime routine and provide practical tips to help you create your own.

A bedtime routine is a series of activities that signal to your body and mind that it's time to wind down and prepare for sleep. It helps create a sense of relaxation and calm, allowing you to transition from the busyness of the day to a peaceful and restful night's sleep.

To start, consider setting a consistent bedtime and wake-up time, even on weekends. This helps regulate your body's internal clock, making it easier to fall asleep and wake up naturally. Additionally, create a sleep-friendly environment by ensuring your bedroom is dark, quiet, and at a comfortable temperature.

Engaging in relaxation techniques before bed can also promote better sleep. This may include activities such as reading a book, listening to soothing music, or practicing gentle stretching or yoga. Avoid stimulating activities such as using electronic devices or watching TV, as the blue light emitted can disrupt your circadian rhythm.

Another crucial aspect of a bedtime routine is limiting caffeine and alcohol intake, especially in the evening. While caffeine is a known stimulant that can interfere with sleep, alcohol may initially make you feel drowsy but can disrupt your sleep patterns later in the night.

Furthermore, consider incorporating exercise into your routine. Regular physical activity has been shown to improve sleep quality and duration. However, it is important to note that intense exercise close to bedtime may have the opposite effect. Aim to finish your exercise sessions at least two to three hours before bedtime.

In conclusion, creating a bedtime routine is a powerful tool to improve your sleep quality. By establishing consistent sleep and wake times, creating a relaxing environment, engaging in calming activities, and being mindful of your caffeine and alcohol consumption, you can set yourself up for a restful night's sleep. Remember, quality sleep is essential for overall health and well-being, and incorporating a bedtime routine into your lifestyle is a small but significant step towards harnessing the sleep benefits of exercise.

The Power of Napping and Power Naps

In our fast-paced world, it seems like there's never enough time to accomplish everything on our to-do lists. With the constant demands of work, family, and social commitments, it's no wonder that many people feel exhausted and burned out. But what if there was a simple and natural way to recharge and boost our energy levels? Enter the power of napping and power naps.

Napping has long been associated with laziness or a lack of productivity. However, research has shown that taking a short nap during the day can actually improve cognitive function, enhance creativity, and increase productivity. In fact, some of the world's most successful individuals, such as Albert Einstein, Leonardo da Vinci, and Winston Churchill, were known to be avid nappers.

So, what exactly is a power nap? It's a brief nap that typically lasts between 10 and 30 minutes. Unlike longer naps, which can leave you feeling groggy and disoriented, power naps are designed to provide a quick burst of energy and mental clarity. They allow your brain to rest and recharge, without entering into the deeper stages of sleep that can leave you feeling groggy upon waking.

The benefits of power napping are numerous. Firstly, napping can improve your mood and reduce stress. Studies have shown that even a 10-minute nap can significantly reduce feelings of fatigue and increase alertness. In addition, napping has been linked to improved memory and learning, as it helps consolidate information and improve recall.

Furthermore, power naps can boost creativity and problem-solving skills. During sleep, the brain processes information and makes new connections, leading to enhanced cognitive abilities. This can be especially beneficial for individuals working on complex tasks or trying to solve challenging problems.

In terms of physical health, napping has also been found to have positive effects. It can reduce the risk of heart disease, lower blood pressure, and improve overall cardiovascular health. Additionally, napping has been shown to enhance the immune system, leading to a stronger defense against illnesses and infections.

In conclusion, the power of napping and power naps cannot be underestimated. By incorporating short periods of rest and relaxation into our daily routines, we can reap numerous benefits for our physical and mental well-being. So, the next time you find yourself feeling tired or overwhelmed, don't hesitate to take a power nap and harness the sleep benefits of exercise to recharge and boost your productivity.

Chapter 9: Conclusion

Recap of the Sleep-Exercise Relationship

In this subchapter, we will summarize the key points regarding the sleep-exercise relationship. Understanding how exercise impacts our sleep is crucial for harnessing the full benefits of both activities and improving our overall health and well-being.

Exercise has been proven to have numerous health benefits, including improved cardiovascular health, weight management, increased muscle strength, and enhanced mental well-being. However, many people overlook the powerful impact exercise can have on our sleep quality. Engaging in regular physical activity can have a positive effect on our sleep patterns and help us achieve a more restful night's sleep.

Firstly, exercise promotes the release of endorphins, which are natural mood enhancers. By boosting our mood and reducing stress levels, exercise can alleviate the symptoms of insomnia and other sleep disorders. Additionally, physical activity increases body temperature, and the subsequent drop in temperature after exercise can signal our bodies to enter a state of relaxation, making it easier to fall asleep.

Moreover, exercise helps regulate our circadian rhythm, the internal clock that controls our sleep-wake cycle. Regular exercise at the same time each day can help establish a consistent sleep schedule, allowing our bodies to anticipate and prepare for sleep, resulting in more efficient and satisfying rest.

Furthermore, engaging in physical activity during the day can reduce the likelihood of experiencing restless legs syndrome or leg cramps at night, common conditions that can disrupt sleep. Exercise also improves overall sleep quality by increasing the amount of time spent in deep sleep, the most restorative stage of the sleep cycle.

It is important to note that while exercise can greatly benefit our sleep, the timing and intensity of our workouts also play a role. Vigorous exercise too close to bedtime may cause overstimulation, making it harder to fall asleep. It is recommended to complete moderate-intensity workouts at least three hours before bedtime to allow the body to wind down.

In conclusion, the sleep-exercise relationship is a mutually beneficial one. Regular exercise not only improves our physical and mental health but also enhances the quality and duration of our sleep. By incorporating exercise into our daily routines, we can experience the full range of health benefits and wake up feeling refreshed, rejuvenated, and ready to take on the day.

Encouragement for Prioritizing Sleep and Exercise

In today's fast-paced world, where we are constantly juggling numerous responsibilities, it can be challenging to find time for ourselves. We often neglect two vital aspects of our well-being – sleep and exercise. However, in order to lead a fulfilling and healthy life, it is crucial to prioritize these two fundamental pillars. This subchapter, titled "Encouragement for Prioritizing Sleep and Exercise," aims to inspire and motivate every individual to make sleep and exercise a priority in their lives.

Regular exercise offers a plethora of health benefits that extend far beyond just physical fitness. Engaging in activities such as jogging, swimming, or yoga not only helps in weight management and cardiovascular health but also boosts mental well-being. Exercise releases endorphins, commonly known as "feel-good" hormones, which enhance mood, reduce stress, and increase overall happiness. Moreover, it improves cognitive function, concentration, and memory, leading to increased productivity and better performance in daily tasks.

Equally important is prioritizing sleep. Sleep is a fundamental biological necessity that restores and rejuvenates our body and mind. It is during sleep that our bodies repair tissues, strengthen the immune system, and consolidate memories. Lack of sufficient sleep not only leaves us feeling fatigued but also weakens our immune system, making us more susceptible to illnesses. Chronic sleep deprivation has been linked to an increased risk of various health conditions, including heart diseases, obesity, and mental health disorders.

By prioritizing both sleep and exercise, we can create a positive cycle that enhances our overall well-being. Engaging in regular physical activity promotes better sleep quality, while quality sleep provides the energy and motivation needed to exercise. Striking a balance between the two is key to leading a healthy and fulfilling life.

To prioritize sleep and exercise, it is important to set realistic goals and make them a non-negotiable part of our daily routine. Start by allocating a specific time for exercise, whether it's in the morning, during lunch breaks, or in the evening. Similarly, establish a consistent sleep schedule, aiming for 7-9 hours of quality sleep each night. Creating a conducive sleep environment, such as keeping the bedroom dark, quiet, and cool, can also improve sleep quality.

In conclusion, prioritizing sleep and exercise is crucial for our overall well-being. By incorporating regular physical activity and quality sleep into our daily routine, we can reap the numerous health benefits they offer. So, let's make a commitment to prioritize sleep and exercise, and witness the positive impact they have on our lives. Remember, a well-rested and physically active individual is more equipped to face life's challenges and enjoy a happier, healthier existence.

Final Thoughts and Next Steps

In this book, we have explored the incredible health benefits that regular exercise can have on our bodies, particularly when it comes to our sleep patterns. We have learned that exercise not only helps us to sweat and burn calories, but it also plays a vital role in improving our sleep quality and duration. By understanding the connection between exercise and sleep, we can make positive changes to our lifestyle that will lead to improved overall health and well-being.

As we conclude this journey, it is important to reflect on what we have learned and consider the next steps we can take to fully harness the sleep benefits of exercise. Firstly, it is crucial to acknowledge that incorporating exercise into our daily routine is not a one-size-fits-all approach. We all have different preferences, abilities, and schedules, so it is essential to find activities that we enjoy and can realistically commit to.

One of the key takeaways from this book is the importance of consistency. Regular exercise, whether it is cardiovascular, strength training, or a combination of both, is vital for reaping the sleep benefits. It is not enough to exercise sporadically; we must strive for consistency in our efforts. This means setting realistic goals and creating a schedule that allows for regular physical activity.

In addition to consistency, it is crucial to listen to our bodies. Pay attention to how exercise affects our sleep. Some individuals may find that working out in the morning energizes them for the day, while others may prefer to exercise in the evening to unwind and promote better sleep. Experiment with different exercise times and styles to determine what works best for us personally.

Furthermore, it is vital to remember that exercise is just one piece of the puzzle when it comes to optimizing sleep. Other factors such as a conducive sleep environment, a consistent sleep schedule, and practicing relaxation techniques before bed all contribute to better sleep. By incorporating these elements into our routine, we can enhance the sleep benefits gained from exercise.

In conclusion, the health benefits of regular exercise are vast, and the impact it can have on our sleep is undeniable. By consistently incorporating exercise into our daily lives, listening to our bodies, and addressing other factors that affect sleep quality, we can truly harness the sleep benefits of exercise. So let's make a commitment to sweat, sleep, and repeat, as we strive towards a healthier and more restful life.

www.ingramcontent.com/pod-product-compliance
Lightning Source LLC
LaVergne TN
LVHW012047070526
838201LV00082B/3829